Aquanatal Exercises

94

Gillian Halksworth

RGN, RM, BA Hons, MN

Books for Midwives Press

Books for Midwives Press is a joint publishing venture
between The Royal College of Midwives and
Haigh & Hochland Publications Ltd

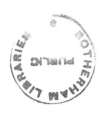

Please note that throughout the book the female personal pronoun has been used in relation to midwives. This is purely for ease of reading and in no way indicates sexism.

Published by Books for Midwives Press, 174a Ashley Road, Hale, Cheshire, WA15 9SF, England

© 1994, Gillian Halksworth

First edition

ISBN 1-898507-05-8

British Library Cataloguing in Publication Data
A catalogue record for this book is available from the British Library

Printed in Great Britain by RAP Ltd

Contents

Acknowledgements

Eternal gratitude is due to many ...

- primarily to my parents for teaching me to swim;
- also to the women who attend and make the sessions so enjoyable;
- and the assistance and modelling for the sketches from Barbara Bale and Domenic;
- artistic help from Paul Watkins;
- the support and advice from Lesley Hobbs and Betty Sweet;
- and, above all the encouragement (nagging!), endless reassurance and belief in me, from Henry Hochland and his team, without whom this would not have been possible!

"I can no other answer make, but thanks and thanks and ever thanks" (Shakespeare)

Dedication

To the members of the Taff Ely Domino Team of Midwives, Pat (who suffered much during the compilation of this book), Jackie, Debbie, Kay, Angie and Linda, all of whom I am privileged to work with and am grateful to for the support, fun and friendship we have shared.

Introduction

This book began with an interest and active involvement in coaching swimming and leading aquanatal classes. Many midwives have asked for assistance and advice in establishing and organizing classes. This book offers answers to most of the main questions which are often raised, as well as exploring some of the literature available and considering various aspects of aquanatal.

It is not intended to be a "complete manual" or an "Aquanatal Made Simple" book. The aim is to provide a basic guide upon which to build, for anyone thinking about undertaking the role of an aquanatal teacher. Neither does it set out the full range of exercises in detail, but simply gives a background and provides examples to facilitate the planning of a suitable aquanatal programme. Guidelines are given to assist in teaching the sessions and encourage high standards of safety. These will promote and facilitate enjoyable sessions for participants and midwives alike.

As this book is aimed at, and has a bias towards, midwifery readership, it assumes that the reader is acquainted with normal anatomy and physiology and the adaptive changes of the human body in pregnancy. Knowledge of normal exercise physiology is also useful (see Wiswell, 1991; Knuttgen and Emerson, 1974).

CHAPTER 1

Why Exercise?

Although it is difficult to analyse conclusively the reasons why people exercise, contemporary attitudes towards fitness, exercise and body image are clearly demonstrated in the proliferation of various exercise programmes.

Artal and Artal Mittlemark (1991) suggest that there is a complex interaction of many variables and an interplay of various motives that determine an individual's behaviour. Some reasons being conscious decisions and others subconscious. Their summary of the reasons is listed below.

1. Sporting activities can offer a means of demonstrating, experiencing and measuring individual achievement and hence improving self-esteem.

2. Exercise can often be used as a diversion tactic to avoid dealing with other problems and conflicts.

3. Enhanced mastery. A feeling of satisfaction when participating in something known to be good for them.

4. Physical exercise is hard work. The sense of feeling good after a hard workout session can provide a feeling of fulfilment.

5. Vigorous exercise can be used as a vehicle whereby anger, stress, frustration and tension can dispersed.

6. Sporting activities are often seen as an opportunity for social interaction and the development of social skills. Experiences gained can lead to an increased sense of team work and team cohesion; exposure to the sense of winning and losing and the competitive and ambitious negotiations present in many sporting activities are useful skills which can be utilized in general life.

Psychologically, therefore, there may be many reasons for undertaking exercise sessions. Furthermore, the Department of Health (1992) suggests that exercise can assist in promoting and maintaining a healthy lifestyle and physical fitness. The World Health Organisation (WHO) state that good health is not only,

> the feeling of mental and physical well being .... also the presence of vigour, vitality and social well being - a zest for living (WHO, 1946).

This definition has been criticised for the idealism portrayed in the statement. It specifies a state which some consider impossible to attain and suggests that we are unhealthy if we do not attain this level of well-being. However, it does provide a basis from which further discussions about health can take place. WHO (1946) depicted physical fitness as,

> being able to carry out daily tasks with vigour . . . and enjoy leisure pursuits and meet unforeseen circumstances.

Fletcher (1991) and Mellion (1985) also suggest that by being physically fit, women can more easily cope with the stresses that life brings, particularly adapting to the role of motherhood. The increase in sense of well being and self-esteem are among the benefits gained from exercise. It is these two areas that are important in facilitating the change in roles that childbirth brings.

Many other scholars advocate the benefits of exercise - the majority of people feeling both psychological and physical benefits, which include weight control, improved self-esteem, prevention of heart disease and prevention of osteoporosis (Fletcher, 1991; Wiswell, 1991; Rutherford, 1990; Wolfe *et al*, 1989; Katz, 1985; Mellion, 1985; Bruser, 1968).

There has certainly been an increase in the uptake of aerobic and exercise programmes, and exercise has become a fundamental part of life for many. When pregnancy is added to life's events, many women are reluctant to forsake the exercise programmes they have embarked upon and the benefits they have gained from them.

Benefits of exercise during pregnancy

The physiological changes in a woman's body during pregnancy are often perceived to inhibit exercise. Certainly, the anatomical changes occurring during pregnancy, such as laxity of joints and ligaments,

2

together with increased weight and the continuing shift in the centre of gravity, may mean that pregnant women are more susceptible to injuries during exercise (Artal *et al*, 1990; 1989).

The physiological changes induced by exercise add to the changes during pregnancy, by increasing the stress on the body. This stimulates the body to make adjustments to accommodate to the demands being made upon it (Wiswell 1991). Muscular exercise increases oxygen requirements and carbon dioxide production of muscle cells and evokes integrated changes in ventilation and haemodynamics. For example, intensive exercise sessions may demand a 20-fold increase in the body's energy output and up to an 8-fold increase in cardiac output. Adjustment is needed by the body to accommodate the increase in heat production during exercise. Fluid and electrolyte balances will be affected and fuel sources depleted. Endocrine and neuromotor activity are increased, as they are intrinsic factors responsible for oxygen extraction and utilization. Oxygen extraction is related to cellular metabolic function and is regulated by enzyme activity and production, as well as fuel availability. Glucose uptake is increased and systemic hypoglycaemia is prevented by increased hepatic glucose production.

In addition to the above-mentioned metabolic changes, other hormonal adaptations include increased glucagon, cortisol, adreno-corticotrophic hormone, growth hormone, epinephrine and norepinephrine levels and decreased insulin levels. At the beginning of an exercise session the initial supply of oxygen is used quickly, leading to an initial "oxygen deficit". Following the exercise session the body restores the muscles energy pool to the pre-exercise state and facilitates the removal of waste products produced from the exercise session. This is often referred to as the "oxygen debt" (Wiswell, 1991).

The extent of the body's adjustment depends on many factors, external as well as internal. Individual aspects such as age, sex, body weight and health status are significant as well as the type and duration of the exercise being undertaken and the environment in which it is performed. Knuttgen and Emerson (1974) found that exercise in pregnancy performed at a steady rate, increased oxygen uptake and the utilization of carbohydrates but there was no evidence of ventilatory impairment or dyspnoea.

There is an increase in endocrine and neuromotor activity; thermoregulation mechanisms need modification, due to heat production. Associated with these are alterations in fluid and electrolyte balance, and energy levels are increased. However, the body normally accommodates and adjusts to this stress and will function normally for different exercise sessions.

Particular benefits have been found to be attributable to exercise training and conditioning, which may well be advantageous to the pregnant woman. Researchers have found a reduction in catecholamine response, and an increase in the capacity of the aerobic system, resulting from exercise training, can assist in preparing women for the physical and psychological stress of labour (Artal Mittlemark, 1991; Russell *et al,* 1984; Rauramo, Anderson and Loatikaimen, 1982).

The efficiency of the cardiovascular system can be improved. Physical training results in an ability to utilize oxygen more efficiently when increased demands are made. This is associated with the heart strengthening, whilst beating more powerfully and more slowly, hence improving an individual's aerobic capacity. Specifically, this enables a pregnant woman to be more prepared for the demands made upon the body during her labour (Cullum and Mowbray 1992; Artal *et al,* 1991; Kulpa, White and Vischer, 1987; Morton, Paul and Metcalfe, 1985; Wilson and Gisolfi, 1980; Dressendorfer, 1978).

Training and conditioning not only increase the cardiopulmonary system but also influence insulin sensitivity in exercising muscles. This increases the capacity to mobilise and oxidize fats, and decreases both the rate of depletion of muscle glycogen during exercise, and secretion of catecholamines.

One study demonstrated positive results in a cohort of 36 multigravida women. They were divided into two groups, one of which was the control. The other group participated in regular exercise programmes whilst pregnant. Both groups were monitored throughout pregnancy. During labour both groups were assessed in terms of pain perception. Samples of blood were taken for levels of ß-endorphin, cortisol, human growth hormone and prolactin. Results revealed an elevation in plasma ß-endorphin in the exercise group. This difference was maintained throughout labour. Pain perception analysis was significantly reduced in the cohort who had exercised. Likewise, there was a reduction in the levels of cortisol, human growth hormone and prolactin levels during labour for the exercise conditioned group (Varrassi, Buzzano and Edwards, 1989).

The researchers suggested that there was an association between ß-endorphin levels and pain perception. In the study, Varrassi, Buzzano and Edwards (1989) demonstrated that physical conditioning during pregnancy increases the ß-endorphin levels, and suggested that this had positive effects on the ability to cope better with labour. The final analysis suggested that exercise conditioning during pregnancy seems to be beneficial in reducing stress levels and pain perception during labour (Varrassi, Buzzano and Edwards, 1989).

Advantages of water exercise

The type of exercise undertaken has different effects on the body. As pregnancy advances, the metabolic cost of any given task increases. Hence, non-weightbearing exercises, which have less metabolic cost, and are potentially less injurious, are suggested as being more suitable during pregnancy (Durak, Jovanovic-Peterson and Peterson, 1990; Sibley *et al*, 1989; Bruser, 1968).

As pregnancy progresses, the physiological changes in the pregnant woman's body may limit her performance and agility in many ways, and affect her choice of exercise programmes. Exercise sessions in water can be enjoyed, as the feelings of weightlessness, freedom and mobility can be used positively to increase physical fitness and improve psychological well-being by enhancing self-esteem. In addition, any concern about thermoregulation during exercise is reduced, as the ability to eliminate heat is greater in water and the potential teratogenic effects caused by a rise in core temperature avoided (Katz, McMurray and Cefalo, 1991).

Since ancient times, the therapeutic properties of water have been recognized and used. Religious rites and practices have used water as symbolic gestures often stemming from its life giving properties (Ezk. 36:25; Matt. 3:11; Eph. 5:26; Rev. 7:17).

These therapeutic practices are continued today. Hydrotherapy is a useful means to maintain and improve suppleness, strength and stamina and is often used for sports injuries. Similarly, swimming is known to be a beneficial physical activity (Harrison, 1993; Reid Campion, 1990; Katz, 1985).

Non-weightbearing exercise performed in water is suggested to be ideal for pregnancy. The risks of injury are slight, provided that a safe programme is planned and individual needs are met (Harrison, 1993; Katz, McMurray and Cephalo, 1991; Sibley *et al*, 1981; Katz, 1985).

Other research undertaken by McMurray *et al* (1988), studied the effect of pregnancy on metabolic responses during rest, immersion and aerobic exercise in water. Using a cohort of 12 women the researchers evaluated the responses of the "fetal-maternal unit" to immersion and exercise in the water at 15, 25 and 35 weeks gestation. Underwater ultrasound visualised fetal body, limb and breathing movements. Although there were changes in the metabolic responses, (plasma cortisol concentrations remained lower during immersion and exercise, triglyceride levels were elevated with exercise and blood glucose levels declined slightly during exercise), these did not have any detrimental effects. The fetal heart rates were within the normal range during the maternal activity. There was no uterine activity seen during the exercise session at 25 or 35 weeks gestation. Maternal temperature and serum alphafetoprotein levels were unaffected at all the stages of the study. The study concluded that immersion and moderate exercise in water do not result in any metabolic compromise. Similarly, maternal and fetal well-being does not appear to be unduly affected.

The authors compared this general lack of effect with results from other studies involving similar levels of exercise on land and found that when the exercise was on land potential problems for the fetus were highlighted (Durak, Jovanovic-Peterson and Peterson, 1990; Jovanovic, Kessler and Peterson, 1985). There was an increase in maternal temperature and a decrease in uterine blood flow, resulting from a decreased plasma volume and shunting of blood to exercising muscles. These factors suggest that there was a change in the fetal heart rate resulting from the land exercise.

McMurray *et al* (1988) comment that the plasma volume expansion with immersion exercise programmes contributes to the normal fetal heart rate responses seen in their study. These results support the hypothesis that water exercises are more beneficial to both mother and fetus than land exercises.

Continuing further in the comparison with land exercise, McMurray *et al* (1988) also found that maternal heart rate responses during immersion in water were less marked. Hydrostatic pressure was thought to be responsible for this. The hydrostatic pressure of water exerts a force which acts uniformly on the body to push extravascular fluid into the vascular space, resulting in a rapid expansion of plasma volume. As the intravascular volume increases, a diuresis is initiated. Renal vascular resistance decreases and hence there is an increase in filtration. The study showed that immersion of women in water for 20-40 minutes results in a 300-400ml loss in fluid, while blood volume is maintained. It is possible that immersion therapy could be used to alleviate symptomatic oedema in some women, however the long-term effects of this relief are not clear (Katz, McMurray and Cephalo, 1991; McMurray *et al*, 1988).

The effects of hydrostatic pressure noted above are particularly related to water aerobic sessions. Whether a similar extravascular fluid redistribution occurs during swimming is not clear. Swimming in a supine position causes some redistribution of fluid volume, but because the body is not totally immersed, the effects of hydrostatic pressure will be less. Most swimmers tend to adopt a vertical position at various times during the exercise session and therefore will benefit from the hydrostatic effect at these periods (Katz, McMurray and Cephalo, 1991).

Harrison (1993) suggests that water exercise is particularly suited to the physically disabled and the overweight person. The pool offers a discreet environment to those feeling ungainly whilst pregnant as their size and shape are not so noticeable in the pool. This reduces their selfconsciousness, as well as enabling exercises to be performed which would be stressful on land, but easily done in water.

Resistance of the water
Resistance occurs when an object moves through a liquid. The frontal resistance depends on the shape of the object, the speed and the density of the fluid. When swimming, resistance is kept to a minimum by streamlining the body. Eddy currents cause turbulence behind objects moving through water, creating a drag, which reduces forward motion. The less streamlined the body, the greater the turbulence (Amateur Swimming Association (ASA), 1985).

Exercises in water can, therefore, be made easier or harder by reducing or increasing resistance. To make the exercises easier, less turbulence is created by reducing the frontal resistance and becoming more streamlined. This reduces the muscular effort required to move through the water and therefore makes exercise easier. To make the exercises harder, the resistance must be increased. It is necessary, therefore, to change the speed and thus increase the turbulence; changing the shape of the body to increase frontal resistance will also ensure increased muscular activity.

Upthrust
When an object is placed within liquid the upthrust effect of liquid is balanced by the downward force of gravity and buoyancy is

achieved. This gives the feeling of weightlessness. Buoyancy can be used to exercise harder in a similar way to resistance (ASA, 1985). Floats can be used to work opposite both the upthrust effect and the force of gravity to increase the utilization of muscular activity.

Psychological benefits of exercising

The psychological benefits of exercising are reported by many as being made up of improved confidence and self-esteem with an associated reduction in depression, anxiety and physical discomfort during pregnancy (Artal and Artal Mittlemark, 1991; Huch and Erkkola, 1990; Wallace *et al*, 1986; Mellion, 1985; Hughes, 1984; Sonstroem, 1984).

Pregnancy is often a challenging and changing time for women. Physically the changes in body image are received positively by some, yet distastefully by others. Psychologically, the new responsibilities and changes in lifestyle that pregnancy brings have similar positive and negative effects.

Artal and Artal Mittlemark (1991) suggest that to enjoy being physically active and exercising ,

> contributes to a sense of well-being, self confidence and greater emotional and physical resilience

Furthermore, they support the view that the increased stamina gained from exercise is beneficial during labour because it can reduce stress levels, which improves pain tolerance and can prepare the woman for the challenges of parenthood (*ibid.*).

Similarly, Sibley *et al* (1981) found that water exercise had many positive benefits in addition to toning and improved physical abilities. These included an improved appetite, better sleep patterns and an increased feeling of well-being. Huch and Erkkola (1990) also suggest that being able to maintain good bodily control and the pleasure derived from active participation has positive psychological benefits.

Main advantages of water exercise

The principal benefits of water exercise are listed below.

- The buoyancy achieved in the water gives support and allows an increased range of movement; water helps suppleness by enabling a full range of movement within a joint; its soothing properties encourage relaxation and give psychological benefits.

- Individuals can work at their own pace.
- Exercise in water carries a minimum risk of straining or injuring joints, as there is a decreased amount of jarring on the joints of the body and the spine.
- Thermoregulation: the risk of maternal hyperthermia, which can be damaging to the fetus (Edwards, 1967; Miller, Smith and Shephard, 1978) is reduced, as heat is dissipated easily in water, and also the possibility of teratogenic effects, caused by a rise in core temperature, is reduced (Katz, McMurray and Cefalo, 1991).
- Cardiovascular capacity is enhanced by being able to utilize oxygen more effectively and efficiently.
- Venous return is increased, which aids circulation. The effects of hydrostatic pressure can have positive effects on oedema and varicose veins.
- Abdominal tone is improved or maintained. The woman's posture improves and the strain on the back is reduced.
- Water resistance builds muscular strength and stamina.
- Social benefits can be derived from joining a class and meeting other people, although the exercises can be performed alone.
- Preparation for labour.
- Maintenance of fitness, despite bodily changes and the encumbrance of pregnancy.

CHAPTER 2

Practicalities of Planning and Organizing a Session

1. Preparation of the midwife

Midwives need to be adequately and appropriately trained in order to take aquanatal classes. Approved courses, organized by midwives and other professionals are often advertised within the midwifery journals. However, having taken a course it may be worthwhile working with a midwife already taking classes, to develop skills and confidence (see later for more details regarding courses and professional issues).

2. Negotiating time to take classes

In view of the proven benefits of aquanatal exercise, midwives working within the NHS should not have any problem convincing managers of the value of running the classes. NHS midwives can, of course, organize and run the classes independently, if they wish, although if it is discussed with the manager and supervisor of midwives, sessions can be advertised within the units if appropriate, and also the supervisors will provide support and encouragement. Equally, midwives working outside the NHS might, out of courtesy, discuss with their supervisor the advantages of offering the classes to NHS clients.

However, despite the benefits that the classes would bring, some managers may wish to know more about the project before they are convinced of its use. Therefore, when approaching managers be well prepared and demonstrate the benefits with research-based evidence. Use documents such as the local strategy and health gain targets, for instance, and find areas where plans are being made at a local level to improve the health of mothers and babies within the community and suggest that the classes may assist in achieving one of the specifications stated. Have facts and figures of the costs ready, both in terms of the members of staff needed and any cost implications of using the pool.

It will be necessary to negotiate the time taken to run classes, in order to meet the needs of both class and midwife. One option is to take the class out of working hours and then claim time back. Alternatively, negotiate to work a shift at a time which includes the duration of the class. For example, on duty from 9.30 a.m. to 5 p.m., the class would be undertaken first and the shift completed in the hospital/ community.

3. Negotiating the use of a pool

It would be ideal to have sole occupancy of the pool for the session, in order to maintain and ensure the privacy of the participants. This will obviously have to be negotiated with the pool manager.

It will be necessary to take stock of the amenities locally. The opportunities vary and include:

* leisure centres;

* school pools (use of these may be restricted during school hours);

* hotel pools (use of these may be restricted during their busy tourist months);

* hospital pools (if fortunate enough to have one!).

Approach them all and discuss the options with the individual pool managers.

4. Paying for use of the pool

Some pools may ask for a booking fee, which can be quite costly, and in some cases prohibitive. The outlay could be recouped by charging the women attending the aquanatal class, but guaranteed attendance numbers are needed to ensure that this is financially viable. Other pools may just charge the women on entry and expect no initial financial outlay. Alternatively, the management team may employ you to take the session and charge the women on admission in order to cover their costs.

Hotel pools may allow you access, providing you use their catering facilities for refreshments after the session, or they may, as above, charge an admission or a booking fee.

Individual arrangements will need to be negotiated. The advantage of leisure centres is that "Passport to Leisure" schemes operate, enabling women on Social Security payments to attend.

5. Accessibility and car parking

Accessibility is an important aspect to consider when choosing a pool. It must be easily accessible by bus, so that everyone is able to attend. Similarly, car parking must be easily available.

6. Creche facilities

Some pools, mainly at leisure centres, have a creche on site, which is obviously useful for those with toddlers.

Postnatal women can bring their babies and leave them in the care of a suitable attendant at the poolside, where the babies can always be in view of their mothers. Should a baby require breast-feeding or other care, the mother can easily leave the pool and attend to her baby. It is essential, therefore, that someone else (midwife, health care assistant or responsible person) is on hand to care for them.

7. Times of sessions

The timing of the sessions may depend on the availability of the pool. However, if given a choice, then try to accommodate the needs of the women. Consideration needs to be given to women who take children to and from school or childminders. This makes 10-10.30 a convenient time to start the class, as it will give them time to take the children before the class commences, and allows them time to enjoy a coffee afterwards before collecting the children at lunchtime. Evening sessions are popular for women at work during the day, and also for those with other children, enabling them to leave the children with their partners or a babysitter. Again, the time of these sessions will depend on the availability of the pool. A good time might be 7-7.30 pm, allowing time for the evening meal and childcare to be organized. Women should be reminded that it is unwise to have a large meal just before aquanatal classes.

Women returning to the class postnatally often find it difficult to organize themselves and their baby for an early morning session, so late morning or afternoon might be the optimum time for such groups.

8. Temperature of the pool

The temperature of the water and air in the pool area is important. Normally, swimming pools are heated at 25°C to 28°C. This may be impossible to change due to the cost implications involved. However, 30°C was found to be the best temperature for exercise programmes, with the air temperature 2-3°C higher (McMurray *et al*, 1988). Immersion for longer periods in cooler water may result in heat loss and discomfort. Exposure to water of less than 28°C will make the women shiver in an attempt to maintain core temperature. Temperatures above 36°C will cause vasodilation and can limit a person's capacity to exercise.

Therefore, the optimum water temperature suggested for immersion exercise is 28-30°C, with the air temperature higher by two or three degrees, if this can be achieved (*ibid.*).

9. Length of a session

This will depend on the fitness levels and requirements of the individuals within the group. An hour-long session would allow 30-45 minutes for the exercise programme, depending on the ability of the group, and also allow approximately 15 minutes relaxation time (Harrison, 1993; Baum, 1991; Hughes, 1989; Reed and Rose, 1985).

10. Dress

Participants may find that wearing a swimsuit with a higher neckline rather than a low-cut one will give better support to the breasts. Alternatively, maternity swimwear with inner support for breasts is ideal, but can often be expensive. A supportive bra or minimum bounce bra with a T-shirt may be preferred by some participants and be less costly.

Midwives may find it useful to wear a lightweight wetsuit which is sleeveless and covers the torso. A wetsuit is ideal for keeping warm when entering or leaving the pool frequently, but it is not an essential item of clothing.

11. Music

Whether or not music is used is really a matter of personal preference. Balaskas and Gordon (1990) suggest that it may be better to follow your own inner rhythms than trying to keep up with the pace of the music. Others suggest that rhythmical movement to music is enjoyed universally and can contribute to the release of endorphins, leading to a feeling of euphoria (Reid Campion, 1990; Baum, 1991). Similarly, moving to keep in time with the beat of the music can aid the effort given to the exercise.

If music is used, a suitable selection must be chosen. Personal tastes influence the decision, but it is important to be sensitive to other peoples tastes. The beat is important and, given that the exercises in water are generally slower than on land, the beat of the music needs to be slightly slower. It is useful to have all the tracks to be used for a session on one tape, so that there will be no need to change the tapes or handle the cassette player with wet hands. However, using one tape can be restrictive to individual needs. A selection of tapes can be taken to the session and changed to give such variety and flexibility as are necessary to meet the needs of the class.

Using a cassette player in a pool area can be dangerous. A circuit breaker must be used if the machine is connected to the mains. However, a battery operated machine would be safer. Use rechargeable batteries to reduce the cost and make sure that the machine is not touched with wet hands.

12. Useful equipment for the class

- Floats - two per class member
- Swim collar for relaxation
- Hand paddles if required for increasing resistance
- Webbed gloves if required for increasing resistance

Stockists and their addresses can be found in the 'Useful Addresses' section at the end of this book, also in any swimming journal.

Fig. 2.1: Examples of equipment

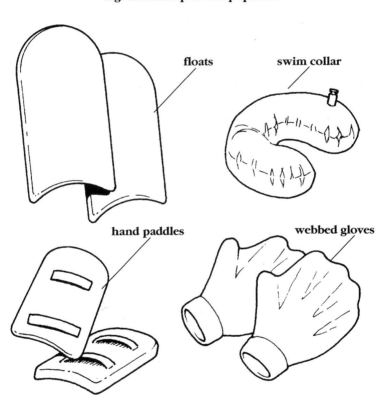

floats   swim collar

hand paddles   webbed gloves

13. Advertising

Promoting the sessions is important. Find suitable places to display posters in hospitals, GP surgeries, libraries and any other pertinent places. Lamination of posters is reasonably priced and will preserve them and enhance their appearance.

Safety aspects

Lifeguard

It is essential to have a lifeguard in attendance when taking the sessions, in addition to the midwife leading the class. It is also useful if the midwives taking the sessions are trained in lifesaving techniques. If sessions are taking place in a public pool then a lifeguard will already be in attendance. It is more discreet to have a female lifeguard on duty if you can, but this may not be possible.

Swimming ability

Identify the swimmers and the non-swimmers within the group.

Health screening

Any health problems should be discussed confidentially before embarking upon the programme and an individual assessment made. Medical problems will often deter people from undertaking any exercise programme at all. During the introductory section it is important to stress that if anyone is attending who has medical problems such as cardiac conditions, pulmonary diseases, metabolic disorders, thyroid problems, back injuries; or any obstetric problems such as hypertension, vaginal bleeding or intrauterine growth retardation then they should make the midwife aware of the situation **before the class commences**. Depending on the problem, it may be necessary to ask them not to participate until a detailed history and discussion with the medical team has taken place (Wallace and Engstrom, 1987).

Similarly, women should not enter the pool if they have an ear, nose or throat infection, an open skin lesion, or a urinary tract infection. Clients should also be advised to avoid exercising if they are recovering from a recent illness, such as influenza or an acute infectious disease.

Environmental factors

The area around the pool is often wet and can be slippery. Care needs to be taken by the women when walking around the area, particularly after the session, when they are readjusting to the weight of pregnancy and the alteration in centre of gravity.

Diving or jumping

Diving or jumping into the pool whilst pregnant is not recommended and should be discouraged.

Socks

It can be useful for the women to wear socks, in order to avoid slipping in the pool itself.

Shallow water

When teaching in shallow water, high impact moves such as jumping during the aerobic section, can cause injuries. Exercises should be adapted accordingly (see section on teaching in small pools).

Avoidance of breast stroke

The effects of relaxation on muscles and ligaments during pregnancy, together with the arching of the lower back in recreational breast stroke (the position usually adopted), can be exacerbated during pregnancy and lead to an increased lordosis. A similar problem can arise with front crawl if the head is held high out of the water. The increased lordosis may potentially lead to back problems, therefore side stroke or back stroke when swimming should be recommended (Reid Campion, 1990; Dale and Roeber, 1987).

Fig. 2.2: Avoidance of recreational breaststroke as it can lead to increased lordosis

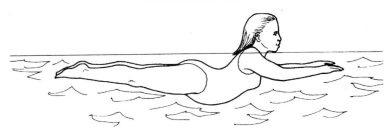

Temperature

Always be aware that the women may be getting cold. Keeping the shoulders under the water will enable them to maintain their body temperature, particularly if the air temperature is cooler. Active sessions of exercise, between slower static exercises help to keep body temperature even. Look for signs of being cold, such as shivering, tenseness and poorly coordinated movements.

Equally, be aware of the women getting too hot. Look for signs of heat exhaustion and fatigue, such as an unusually flushed complexion, nausea, tiredness and dizziness.

Pain or discomfort

Advise the women that if they have any discomfort or pain they should slow down or stop and discuss the problem with the midwife. The exercises should be comfortable to perform. If the women feel any nausea or dizziness they should stop and take a rest.

Adequate space

Ensure that the women are well spaced out so that the exercises can be performed without danger to others. Any floating exercises or free standing exercises must be done at a suitable distance from the pool side to avoid risk of injury.

Demonstrations

When demonstrating any exercises from the side of the pool the midwife must be careful not to slip and should use a non-slip mat.

Size of class

Keeping the class to sensible numbers enables everyone to benefit equally from it and ensures safety. Ideally, there should be 10-15 in each class. This allows an easy rapport to be established. Up to 20 is a manageable number but larger classes than this can be difficult. It may be advantageous to split the class, if the size of the pool and staffing levels permit, and have two sessions running concurrently.

Teaching in small pools

Small pools are often all that is on offer, as leisure centre managers prefer to have these used for water exercise classes, thus keeping the main pool open to the public. Although small pools are often ideal because the water temperature is higher, the depth of the water, however, can be off-putting and restrictive. Non-swimmers, however, may find either the small pool or the shallow end of a larger pool reassuring.

In order to keep as much of the body immersed as possible in the shallower water, many exercises must be performed in a squatting position, or some in a kneeling position. An effective session can still be achieved by increasing resistance; change direction quickly in the water and work against the force of the water as a good first step. Using floats or paddles also increases resistance and adds to the workload, which aids muscular activity and hence adds to the effect of training.

Postnatally, jumping-type exercises, which can be dangerous on land, are safer in water as there is no hard impact with the floor because the buoyancy of deeper water counteracts the landing force. However, in shallow water this is reduced. Frog jumps (either on the spot or travelling through the water) can be undertaken safely by jumping *through* the shallower water, not out of it, by breaking the weight of the body against a float. This is done by pushing down with both hands on the float, so that the body weight is supported by the resistance of the float being forced against the water. Similarly, jumping forwards and backwards through the water, while "scooping" the water in towards the body with the float, will also break the impact and protect the joints from damage.

Tips on teaching aquanatal classes

Voice projection
The instructor must speak clearly, slowly and loud enough for everyone to hear. Be aware that acoustics are often poor in swimming pools and simply raising the voice does not always overcome this problem. Speaking in a monotone becomes boring and thus ineffective. The pitch should be varied to create a lively and enjoyable atmosphere, which can be motivating or relaxing accordingly.

Teaching position
The instructor should be able to see all the women easily, so that help can be given as required. This is easier if the instructor stands on the side of the pool. However, demonstrations of the aerobic session need to be performed from within the pool to avoid risk of injury to the instructor. It might be useful, therefore, to have two midwives at a class.

Demonstrations
Demonstrations indicating limb movements can be given by the midwife standing on the pool side. It is important that they are accurate and should be seen from various viewpoints, so that the women not only see, but understand, the teaching points. The best position for demonstrations will depend on the size and arrangement of the class and the acoustics of the pool.

When demonstrating from the side of the pool, the women can form a semicircle facing the midwife, which will promote a good rapport and a feeling of individual attention. It will also enable everyone to see and hear the instructor. When a particular limb movement is being demonstrated from the side of the pool, a mirror image is created. Therefore, be aware that when demonstrating with the right arm when facing a class, they will naturally use their left arm!

Demonstrations of the warm-up exercises and stretching can be performed from the side of the pool.

Synchronization

Synchronization within the group, i.e. using the same limb or going the same way if moving, and having the appropriate individual space, avoids accidents.

Variety

Progression and variety in the content of the class is required to maintain interest and benefit. Changing the speed of a movement, including variety in content and speed, and the use of different starting positions will all help to achieve this. Also include movement on the spot and travelling through the water, across or up and down the pool.

Exercises can be linked to childbirth. A focus on the breathing techniques for laboour, muscle strengthening for legs in preparation for squatting, pelvic floor muscle exercises for toning and strengthening are all appropriate.

Assessment of the pool

The individual aspects of the pool should be assessed. Some pools have gradients and/or steps, which can be used for some exercises. Look at the most suitable way of using the pool when using travelling exercises, i.e. moving through the water either across or up and down the pool.

Assess the depth of the pool. In order to gain the desired effect from training, it is necessary to work the water hard. The wall of water in front of the body gives greater resistance. Ideally, therefore, the water should be at least waist height, if not deeper. However, as already discussed, adequate depth of water may not always be available (see section on Teaching in small pools).

Timing of exercises

It is important to remember when planning a session that movement in water is slower than on land and therefore time must be allowed for a change of direction or movement.

CHAPTER 3

The Programme

The exercise programme should be arranged to allow the development of stamina, strength and suppleness. The structure of the programme is:

•	warm-up and static stretches	8-10 mins
•	muscular strength and endurance	10-12 mins
•	aerobic and stamina	10-12 mins
•	stretching and cool down	10-12 mins
•	relaxation	10-15 mins

All timings are approximations.

The muscular strength/endurance and the aerobic/stamina section can be altered in order. Harrison (1993) suggests that by having the order as shown above, with aerobics in the middle, assists the maintenance of body temperature and stops the women from getting too cold. They may get cold when aerobics follows the warm-up section, as the following structure of the class will be more static, and may require more warming activities.

Posture, breathing and pelvic floor muscle exercises are basic aspects that should be stressed and encouraged throughout the exercise session.

Basic posture

'Basic posture' is the starting position for most of the exercises, and is referred to throughout the book. The basic posture that should be adopted during any of the upright exercises is as follows:

a)   shoulders should be rounded backwards and down, head lifted tall, neck extended and chin tucked in;

b)   muscles of the abdomen and buttocks should be tightened and drawn in, which stabilises the back, the pelvis should be tucked under, giving a feeling of flattening and extending the lumbar spine;

c)   knees should not be locked back, but maintained in a soft, slightly bent position;

d)   feet should be a comfortable hip distance apart, toes facing forwards, body weight evenly distributed through both legs.

One way of demonstrating and practising the correct posture is to stand with your back against the pool side wall, with your lumbar spine pressed into the wall and knees bent. Standing up tall and straightening the legs more, will give the correct pelvic tilt and the abdominal muscles will be used to support the position.

Breathing patterns

A normal breathing pattern should be maintained during the exercise session. Participants often forget to breathe whilst concentrating on an exercise, so a gentle reminder to continue breathing throughout the exercises is useful! Failure to breathe properly could result in the Valsalva effect, where a pressure is created in the chest with an associated increase in blood pressure, which can lead to a decreased blood supply to the brain, which results in fainting. This can occur in sporting activities when a weight is lifted, or during the straining part of an exercise if the breath is held at the same time. This *should* not occur in aquanatal classes, but it is important to be aware of the possibility and educate women about correct breathing techniques.

To ensure correct breathing techniques are employed, clear explanations must be given. An example is given below.

1.   Exhaling during an active phase of the exercise and inhaling on the relaxation phase, is a simple way of remembering how to breathe correctly.

2.   "Breathing in through the nose as if smelling a hot dinner and exhaling through the mouth as if blowing the dinner to cool it down".

Pelvic floor exercises

Pelvic floor exercises are essential and should be included within the exercise programme both antenatally and postnatally. Wielsen (1988) demonstrated that, following delivery, women who had exercised during pregnancy found that their pelvic floor muscles were stronger in comparison with those in the control group. In addition, muscles toned antenatally stretch and contract more efficiently, which is an added advantage during labour.

Explaining the relevance of these exercises to the women will not only encourage them to exercise postnatally but also continue exercising this important group of muscles for the rest of their lives. The aim is to strengthen the muscles both antenatally and postnatally, which will ultimately prevent long-term problems of stress incontinence or other urinary problems, as well as preventing a prolapse of the pelvic structures, due to a weakness of the pelvic floor. Strengthening these muscles is also said to enhance sexual experiences (Comfort, 1991).

Pelvic floor muscle exercises should be incorporated into the exercise programme and at any additional spare interval, both antenatally and postnatally. One way of describing this particular exercise is to suggest the following, whilst maintaining the basic posture as described above.

- Draw the buttocks together, and the muscles at the front as if you are stopping yourself going to the toilet.
- Then draw the muscles up inside as if it is a lift going up the shaft, first floor, second floor, third floor.
- Hold the muscles there for 3-5 seconds.
- Then let the lift down slowly, as some people want to get off at the second floor, first floor and the ground floor.
- Relax for 2-3 seconds.
- Repeat the exercise a few times slowly and then repeat the exercises quickly.

Gilpin *et al* (1989) and Wiswell (1991) suggest that performing these particular exercises at the two different speeds will improve the muscle tone further. The quicker action provides sufficient intensity to involve recruitment of the "greater tension producing glycolytic fast-twitch" muscle fibres which has beneficial effects in terms of enhancing muscle tone (Wiswell, 1991).

CHAPTER 4

Warm-up Exercises

It is essential to start with a warm-up period. The aims of these warm-up exercises are to prepare the body for the ensuing exercise session and help prevent injuries, such as sprains and muscle tears.

Aims and objectives

1. When initially immersed in water, there is a drop in body temperature. A warm-up period is important. A gradual increase in the body temperature is important as muscle efficiency is enhanced and injuries to muscles avoided.
2. The warm-up period ensures a gradual increase in the blood supply to the muscles and joints. This, in turn, improves the oxygen supply available and results in an increase in the muscle elasticity which reduces muscle viscosity. This improves the tone of the muscle and reduces the risk of injury. Similarly, an increase in the supply of synovial fluid enables an increase in the range of movement, and reduces the stress on the joints.
3. The cardiovascular system is gradually prepared for more strenuous exercises, such as those in the aerobic section.
4. The warm-up also includes some stretching, especially the large muscles, which will be used in the aerobic and strength sections of the exercise programme.

A gradual response by the body to the exercise session should ensure little discomfort and facilitate physical efficiency. The length of the warm-up period will vary from 5-10 minutes. It should include exercises that gradually warm, mobilise and loosen the muscles and joints, increasing the heart rate and body temperature, and incorporate some static stretching exercises.

Leading the warm-up session

- Maintaining correct posture is important throughout the exercise programme and should be stressed during the warm-up period.
- Ensure that the women are using the water to every advantage by having the water covering their shoulders.
- The exercises should not be too intense or fast and should gradually increase the heart rate. They should gently build up in intensity, and work through the body systematically.

Examples of some warm-up exercises

Head and neck

Any movements in this area should be slow and controlled. They should also take place after the shoulders have been loosened. Neck rolls will encourage deep breathing exercises. However, it is important not to drop the head backwards to look at the ceiling as this can be too stressful for the cervical joints and can lead to injury. The exercises in this area should be either turning the head to one side and back to the centre; or allowing the chin to rest on the chest, roll the head from one side to the other, without going backwards.

Mobilising the shoulders and upper spine

Ensure basic posture is adopted (see section on Basic posture at the beginning of Chapter 3), keeping the shoulders under the water. Any of the following can be performed:

- shoulder lifts;
- shoulders drawn forwards and then taken backwards;
- bending the arms with the hands resting on the shoulders, lifting up and down, followed by rotating the elbows in circles forwards and backwards together and then alternately;
- arm swinging;
- keeping the arms straight and out to the sides, drawing circles in a clockwise direction, then anticlockwise, and then in the shape of a figure of eight.

Fig. 4.1: Mobilising the shoulders - lifting and rotating the elbows

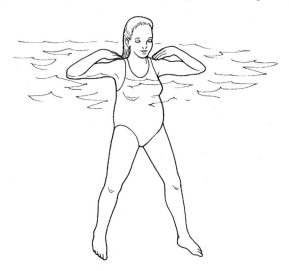

For rotation of the spine, adopt basic posture, take arms in front of the body at shoulder height and rotate from side to side, keeping the hips facing forwards, moving only the torso and head as if looking behind.

Fig. 4.2: Mobilising the upper spine - rotation

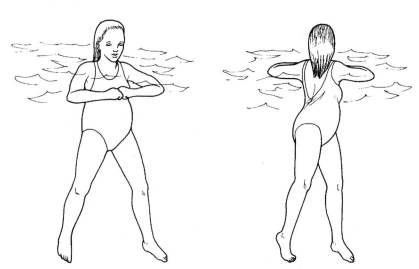

Elbows

There are various exercises for the elbows, some suggestions are shown below.

(a)   Have arms bent in front of the body, fingertips touching the shoulders, bending and stretching forwards.

(b)   Arms out to the sides, palms facing upwards, bending to touch the shoulders and then stretching out to the sides.

(c)   Palms facing downwards, bending and stretching underneath so that the fingertips touch axilla.

(d)   Stretch the arms out and then bring across the body in a hug position.

Fig. 4.3: Elbow exercises

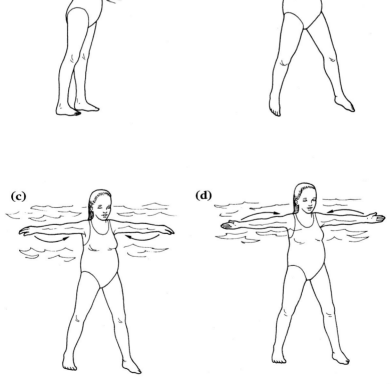

Hands and wrists

With arms outstretched, circle hands forwards and backwards; lift hands upwards and downwards, flexing upwards and pointing downwards.

Rotation of spine and pelvis

Side bends, promoting lateral flexion. Adopting basic posture of pelvis tucked under and abdomen drawn in, shoulders back and down, knees slightly bent.

- Arms out straight to the sides and leaning from side to side stretching further each time.
- Hands on hips, bending slowly to the side, remembering not to lean forwards or backwards.
- Straight arms stretching slowly down the leg to each side.

For pelvic tilts, adopt basic posture, keeping knees slightly bent, with hands either on hips or resting on the side of the pool, draw the pelvis under, hold and relax. Repeat. Then rotate pelvis in a circle or a figure of eight. The movement and stretching should be from the pelvis and spine.

Fig. 4.4: Rotation of spine and pelvis - pelvic tilts and circles

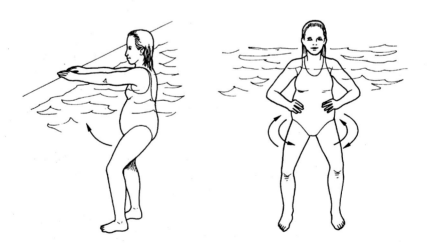

Hips

Resting with one hand on the side of the pool, keeping the arm straight, balance with the other arm straight out to the side. With the weight of the body supported by the leg closest to the pool side, swing the other leg forwards and backwards; follow by drawing circles and then figures of eight with the leg and foot. Turn around and change legs repeating the same exercises.

Fig. 4.5: Hip exercises - leg swings

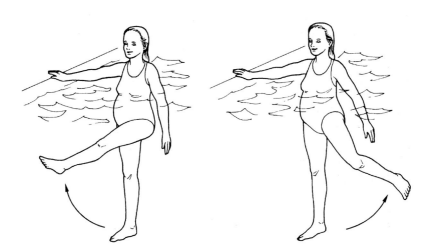

Knees

Resting with one hand on the pool side for balance, weight evenly distributed, basic posture adopted, squat slowly down and stretch up; follow by gentle slow alternate knee lifts; then lift one knee and hold leg behind the body, then bend and stretch the leg.

Ankle

Basic posture, resting with one hand on the side of the pool for balance, the other hand can be resting on hip or extended, circle ankle joint around clockwise and anticlockwise.

These are only a few examples of warming-up exercises, there are many variations of these. Ensuring good posture and incorporating breathing exercises is essential for a warm-up session. Variation prevents boredom for both the women and the midwife leading the session. Gradually increase the pace of this part of the session as the women gradually loosen and warm-up.

CHAPTER 5

Static Stretches

Static stretches, which also assist in the warm-up, enable the muscles to stretch more easily during the ensuing exercise programme. Muscles and joints are protected from injury by the stretch reflex. If a movement is sudden or jerky, the stretch reflex will contract the muscle tissue, preventing any further stretching and inhibiting movement, thereby protecting the muscle and joint from injury.

By performing the stretch in a slow controlled manner, easing into the stretch to a point where it is comfortable and not painful, the tension in the muscle relaxes and the stretch can be taken further. The stretch should be felt in the central part of the muscle and should not be painful. Ultimately this will increase the range of movement and flexibility, enabling the body to perform more efficiently.

Once the muscles have started to warm up, the later part of the warm-up session should involve static stretches, performed slowly in a controlled manner, holding the stretch for 5-10 seconds in this part of the session. Examples are described below.

Examples
Calf and hamstring stretches
CALF STRETCH

- Adopting basic posture, hold on to the side of the pool for support if required. Forward lunge position: with one foot approximately 12" in front of the other, toes pointing forwards, and keeping the back leg straight with the heel of the foot on the floor, and the front leg bent, lean slightly forwards taking most of the body weight on the front leg, until the stretch (not pain!) is felt in the calf of the rear leg. Hold for 5-10 seconds.

Fig. 5.1: Calf stretches - forward lunge position

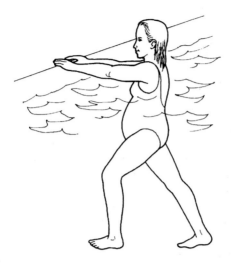

- Following this, lean forwards with hands resting on the front leg above the knee and straighten the leg behind. The stretch should be felt in the back of the thigh in the rear leg. Hold for 5-10 seconds.

Fig. 5.2: Calf stretches

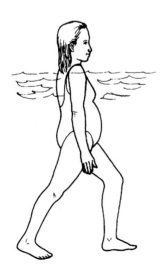 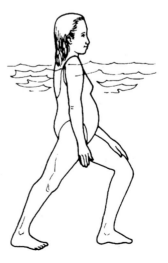

- Bending both legs, bring the back leg in slightly towards the leg in front. Straighten the forward leg, keeping the rear leg bent. The stretch should be felt further down in the calf of the rear leg. Hold for 5-10 seconds.

- Change legs and repeat all the above on the other leg.

OTHER CALF AND HAMSTRING STRETCHES

- Adopting basic posture and holding on to the side of the pool for balance if required, bend one knee up to the chest and support with arm.

Fig. 5.3: Other calf and hamstring stretches

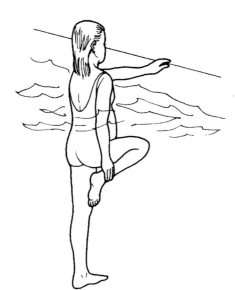

- Using the wall of the pool or graduated steps, keeping one leg bent and supporting the weight of the body, take the other leg to the wall of the pool or rest on one of the steps, keeping the foot flat. Lean forwards towards the leg and feel the stretch in both the calf and hamstring (Fig. 5.4).

Fig. 5.4: Other calf and hamstring stretches

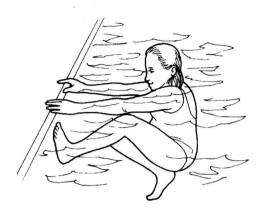

Quadriceps

Adopt basic posture whilst standing with weight evenly distributed. Rest with one hand on the side of the pool for balance, if necessary. Bend one leg behind, with heel pointed towards buttocks. Hold ankle with hand, keeping knees together and pelvis tucked under, abdominal muscles drawn in. Avoid overarching of the back. Hold and repeat with other leg.

Fig. 5.5: Quadriceps

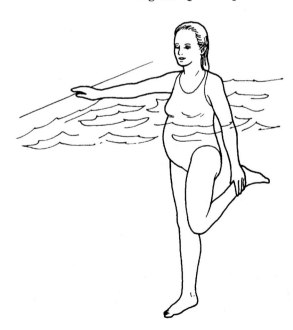

Shoulder and pectoral stretch

- Adopt basic posture. Do shoulder stretches by taking alternate arms upwards and stretching high; then lift arms together and hold.

Fig. 5.6: Shoulder and pectoral stretch

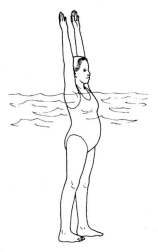

- Take both hands behind the body, and clasp them together, easing and stretching upwards and backwards as far as is comfortable. Postnatally, this may be too uncom–fortable to perform if the breasts are full and painful.

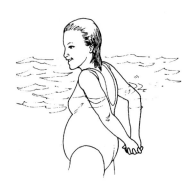

Elbows should not be locked.

Triceps

Stretch one arm above the head close to the ear. Drop the fore arm and hand behind the head, using the opposite arm hold the elbow of the bent arm and pull towards the head, feeling the stretch in the triceps muscle.

**Fig. 5.7: Triceps stretches - standing (in a large pool) and kneeling
(in a small pool)**

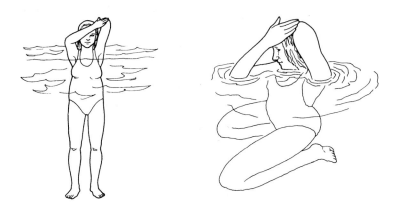

Groin stretches

- Adopting basic posture, slide one leg out to the side, keeping
  both feet flat on the floor, let the other knee bend. The stretch
  takes place in the groin area. Further stretching can be achieved
  by lifting the outstretched leg, depending on the individual.

Fig. 5.8: Groin stretches

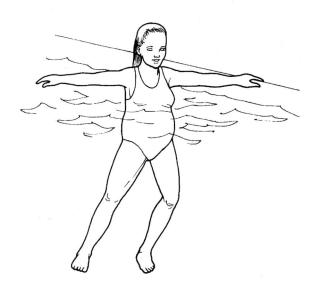

- Alternatively, rest with one arm on the side of the pool for support. Balance on one leg, foot parallel to the wall, and slowly bend the other leg. With the sole of the foot resting against the thigh of the opposite leg, hold the ankle and feel the stretch in the groin. **Note that the foot of outstretched leg should be pointing forwards and the whole foot on the floor.**

Fig. 5.9: Groin stretches

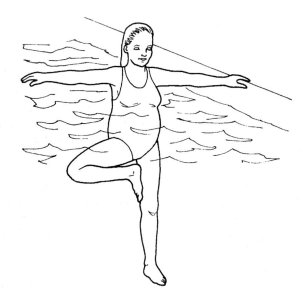

CHAPTER 6

Muscular Strength and Endurance Section

Aims and objectives

a)   To improve the condition of ligaments and tendons, which in turn improves body shape as muscles tone and become firmer.

b)   To increase muscular strength, and thus an improvement in posture, which in turn lessens the strain on the spine.

c)   To improve stamina enabling an individual to participate in a physical activity for longer and with less tiredness.

This section of the programme is "isotonic exercise", which promotes a full range of movement whilst building strength. There are two types of muscle contraction incorporated within this: eccentric, which produces a lengthening of the muscle; and concentric, which produces a contraction and shortening of the muscle.

There is a difference in the way muscles are used when comparing work within water and on land. When exercising on land, eccentric muscle work is common, as this balances the effects of gravity. However, exercise programmes within water are mostly concentric muscular action, working against the resistance of the water. For example, when bending the arm on land it is the shortening of biceps muscle which acts as the prime mover. When extending this arm out again it is the effect of gravity and control of the biceps muscle in an eccentric contraction, with the muscle fibres gradually lengthening, which allows the arm to return to the extended position. However, in water, the triceps muscles are more active in this movement as the resistance of the water causes a concentric contraction of the tricep muscle to extend the arm once again.

It is this work against the resistance of the water that aids the strengthening process and is an important aspect to consider in planning any of the exercise programme, with particular reference to this section.

Teaching points

- When teaching this section it is useful to coordinate the routine around the three main areas of the body: upper, middle and lower.

- Similarly, when planning a routine, make it easy to change from one exercise to another, so that the session runs smoothly. If using equipment (such as floats), use it for the whole routine to prevent any unnecessary disruptions.

- Ensure that the group adopts the correct posture and performs the exercises properly.

- There should be a progressive development to ensure that muscles are strengthened and stamina built. However, it is important that individuals participate at their own level and so development can only be considered on an individual basis.

- Repetition of the exercises aids the development of the muscular strength aimed for. These exercises could be repeated between 8 and 16 times, depending on the fitness of the group. Eight repetitions works in quite well with the music and repetitions can be built around this number to meet the needs of the group. Alternatively, a short planned routine can be repeated, rather than individual exercises.

Examples

Upper body - triceps and biceps

These exercises are aimed at strengthening the muscles of the arms, shoulders and spine.

Fig. 6.1: Triceps and biceps - bending both arms together and alternately

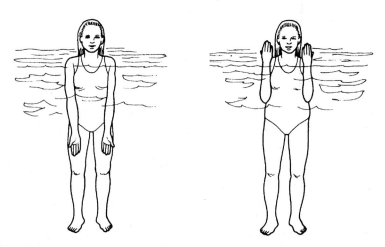

i) Adopt basic posture. Ensure that the water is over the women's shoulders. Arms should be extended downwards with the backs of the hands resting on the thighs. Keeping wrists and hands straight, bend both arms together as quickly and forcefully as possible to touch the shoulders and straighten the arms back to touch the thighs. Repeat. Then perform the same with alternate arms.

ii) Similar posture, with arms stretched out to the sides, backs of the hands uppermost. The upper arm remains still and the lower arm is slowly bent down from the elbow and a slow controlled movement as the arms are stretched out again. Repeat. Floats can be added to increase resistance, to strengthen biceps and triceps.

iii) Alternatively, check posture, and using floats, push down vertically as quickly as possible and as slowly as possible as the float rises. This can either be done with one float, or with one in each arm together and alternately. Similarly, one can be held between the two hands, one hand uppermost the other underneath, and pushed down and released slowly.

Fig. 6.2: Triceps and biceps - pushing down vertically

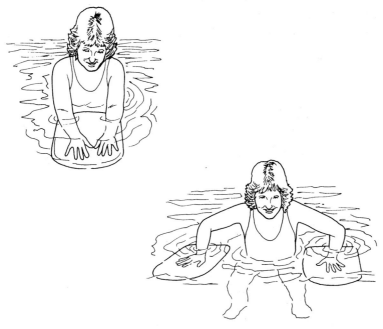

Upper body - pectoral muscles

iv)   Adopt basic posture. Ensure water is over the womens' shoulders. The arms should be bent as if praying, but hands clenched. The arms should be taken out to the side at shoulder height, keeping arms under the water, and returned. Repeat. To develop strength these can be performed faster, and add further resistance with floats in each hand or webbed gloves.

Fig. 6.3: Pectoral muscles

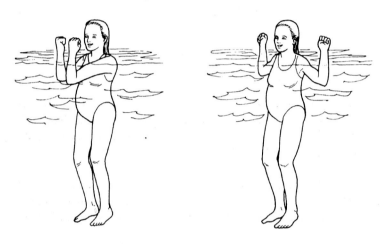

Rotation of the spine can be incorporated here by alternating arms across the body and then away from the body.

Fig. 6.4: Rotation of spine - kneeling (in a small pool)

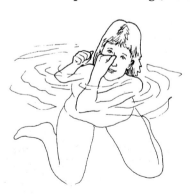

v)   Adopt basic posture. Spread feet wide apart. With arms stretched out to the side, bend one knee and stretch out further to this side. Swing the arm back through the water to the middle and change sides, bending the knee on the opposite side and stretching out to this side. Repeat equal times on each side.

vi) In a similar position but with hands and arms by the sides, slowly bend sideways at the waist and reach down the leg. Only the torso should move, the hips remaining static. Repeat both sides. Floats or webbed gloves can be used with both these exercises.

Middle body

These exercises are aimed at strengthening the spine and abdominal muscles.

Using floats, one under each arm for support, lie back and allow the body to float. It is important when performing these exercises both antenatally and postnatally that the rectus muscle has been assessed (see Postnatal chapter).

i)   Bend both knees together to a comfortable position near the abdomen. Keeping the legs touching, twist both knees over to one side and then to the other. Repeat 10-15 times each side.

Fig. 6.5: Abdominal muscles - twists

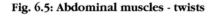

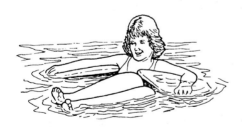

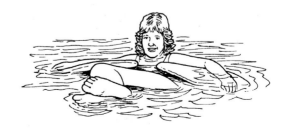

ii)   Curls. This is particularly strengthening for the straight
        abdominal muscles. Stretch both legs out straight on the surface
        of the water, keeping the toes out of the water as far as
        possible. Slowly bend both knees towards the chest.

Fig. 6.6: Abdominal muscles - curls

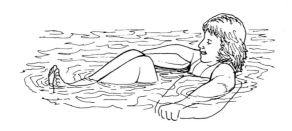

iii)   Alternate knee to chest, straightening one whilst bending the
        other in a slow controlled manner.

Fig. 6.7: Alternate knee to chest

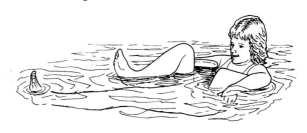

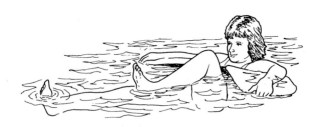

iv)   Curls and twist. Bend both legs to the chest and twist over to
        the side, stretching the legs out to the side. Bend and bring
        the legs in again to the chest and twist to the other side and
        repeat.

v)   Scissor and 'V's. Open the legs out wide into a 'V' shape and back together again keeping the legs close to the surface of the water. Repeat 10 times. Then, when bringing the legs together again, extend further over, crossing the legs as if they are a pair of scissors. Then open wide and cross the other way. Repeat.

vi)   Straight leg kicks up and down into the water rather than through the water, as in crawl stroke, but in a slow and controlled manner.

vii) Rolls. While floating, bring the knees up to the baby or chest, toes out of the water. In this position tilt forward into a vertical position and stretch both legs out behind, so that women will now be floating on their stomachs. Reverse the roll back and repeat.

Fig. 6.8: Abdominal muscles - rolls

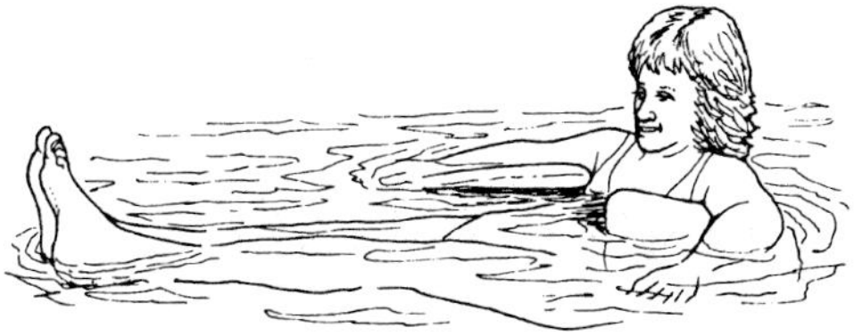

(a) Legs extended

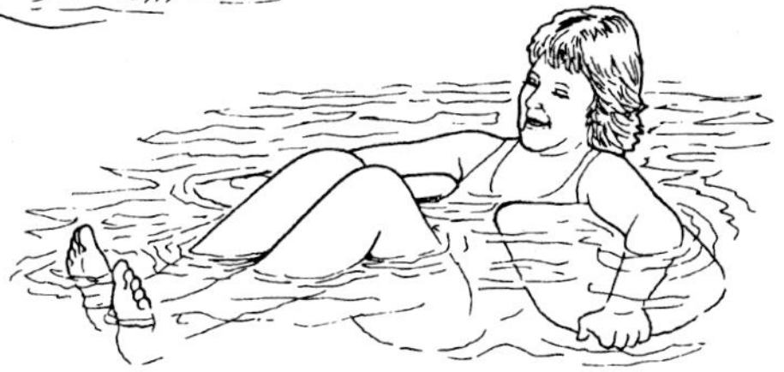

(b) Bring knees to abdomen

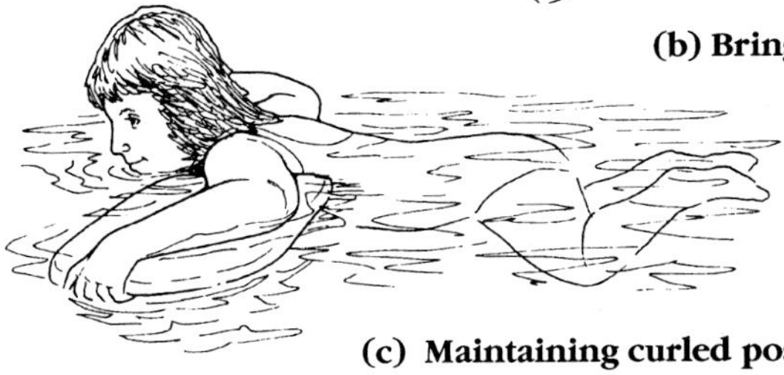

(c) Maintaining curled position, roll forwards

(d) Extend the legs and stretch out. Then curl again and roll back the other way into the starting position.

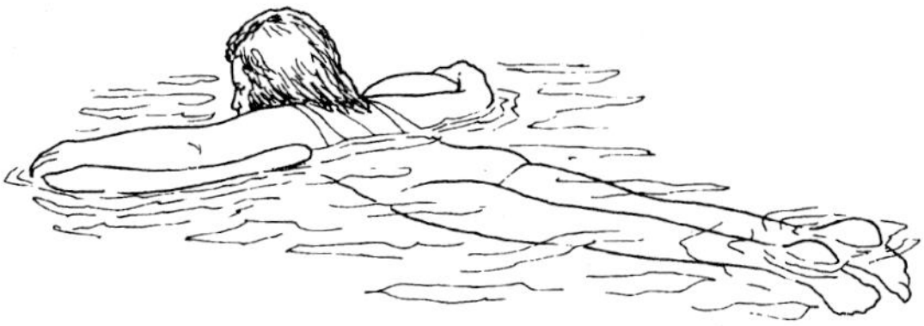

Lower body

These exercises are aimed at strengthening the areas of pelvis, thighs and lower legs.

i)   Pelvic floor exercises can be undertaken at this point (see section on Pelvic floor exercises).

ii) Squats for strengthening thighs. Stand in waist-high water, either facing the pool side with both hands resting on the side of the pool or standing adjacent to the pool side, with one hand resting on it . Adopt basic posture with feet wide apart. Squat down into the water, in a slow and controlled manner, keeping the torso vertical and the pelvis tilted under. Slowly stand up again, ensuring a good stretch on rising from the squat. Repeat, easing the squat deeper, if possible.

There are many exercises that can be performed to tone the lower legs and a few examples are given below.

iii) Leg raises. Hold on to the side of the pool, standing in a comfortable depth of water. Adopt basic posture, facing the pool side. Stand on one leg, keeping the torso still. Slowly lift the other leg out to the side and back to the middle. Repeat with each leg. Then repeat performing cross over scissor actions either in front of, or behind the static leg.

iv) Turn to stand at right angles to the pool side so that leg lifts forward and backwards can be performed. These can be done with each leg. Follow by figure of eight movements with a straight leg.

v)   Knee lifts can also be performed in this position. Adopt basic posture and raise leg with knee bent to a comfortable position. Bring the foot slowly back to the floor. Repeat on both sides.

vi) Following knee lifts, hip rotations can be undertaken. Lift leg with knee bent and move the leg from the hip joint across the body, the torso remaining stationary.

vii) Bottom kicks can also be performed in this position. Bend the leg behind, as if to touch the buttocks, in a slow and controlled manner. Repeat on both sides.

viii) For progression, in the same position, allowing the knee to bend and hip to twist, draw a figure of eight with the leg in this bent position.

ix)   Stork walk. Adopt basic posture in waist-high water. Clasp hands behind the back. Raise the knee to a comfortable height. Maintaining posture and not leaning forward, straighten the leg out in front of the body. Hold for a few seconds before bringing the foot down to the floor. Walk forward with the movement. Repeat, walking across the pool.

Fig. 6.9: Stork walk

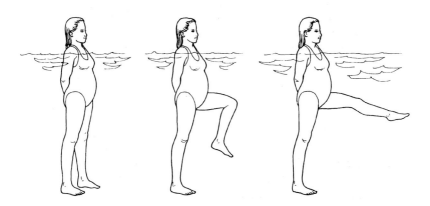

CHAPTER 7

Aerobic or Stamina Section

Aims and objectives
•   To produce a training effect to develop fitness in the cardiovascular system.
•   To improve the capacity and efficiency of the cardiovascular system, in terms of delivering oxygen to the muscles and eliminating waste products.

The definition of aerobics is 'with oxygen'. In exercise programmes 'aerobics' refers to the type of activity, during which the muscles of the body convert stored fuel into energy in the presence of oxygen. A less efficient, and yet possible, way of achieving this is by the anaerobic (without oxygen) action of muscles. However, this results in a rapid build up of waste products, such as lactic acid, which can restrict the length of time the muscle can go on working efficiently. It can also cause muscle cramps and stiffness.

By improving the capacity and efficiency of both circulation and respiratory systems the oxygen supply to muscles will improve, and any waste products produced from muscular activity will be eliminated more efficiently. The exercises should improve the body's ability to absorb large amounts of oxygen, transport it efficiently to tissues via the blood, and produce energy enabling the muscles to work effectively.

During the aerobic sessions the exercises should progressively develop in intensity. Basic posture should be emphasized as always. It should be an enjoyable and fun part of the session!

Teaching points
The choice of exercises for this section are many and varied. Partner and group work can be incorporated as well as swimming. Monitor the fitness level of the group and adapt exercises to meet their needs.

Examples of aerobic exercises

i)   Adopt basic posture. Rest hands on the hips initially. Lift alternate knees up to a comfortable position, in an exaggerated marching movement. Slowly at first, gradually increasing in speed. Keep the rhythm going with the legs. Use the arms, either in a cycling movement as if running, or as in the pectoral muscle exercises earlier, with elbows bent in a praying position and hands clenched. Keeping arms vertical, take them out to the side of the body, at right angles to it. Other arm movements to do with this exercise could be: stretching up to the sky; alternating with the leg movement; punching the water as if boxing; or, "canoeing", using both arms on the same side as the leg is lifted, scooping the water past the body in a sweeping action, really heaving the arms through the water. Repeat on the other side. Postnatally, these can be developed to alternate knee lifts to elbow, and alternate hand to heel. Also, kicking the heels to the rear. Alternatively, this exercise could lead on to stride jumps, with feet apart, alternating arms with legs, jumping as you cross legs in stride jumps. (See section on 'Teaching in small pools'.)

ii) Use floats to take the weight of the body. Adopt the basic posture, with knees bent in a squatting position.

Fig. 7.1: Aerobic exercises - basic posture with knees bent

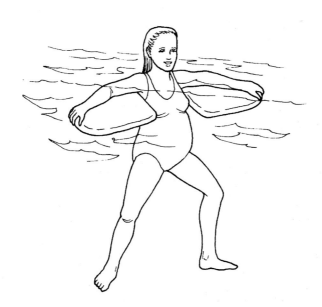

Lift alternate legs to the side as if rocking initially, increase in speed, bouncing in between changing legs.

Fig. 7.2: Aerobic exercises - leg lifts

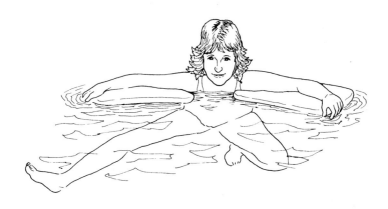

Once the rhythm is established, alternate legs can be straightened, as if performing a Russian dance. Using the floats for balance, the stretch can be taken further on the opposite side to that of the legs. The direction of the legs can be changed to alternate leg stretches and then kicks forward, with alternate arms with floats, similar to an exaggerated march.

Fig. 7.3: Aerobic exercises - leg stretches and kicks

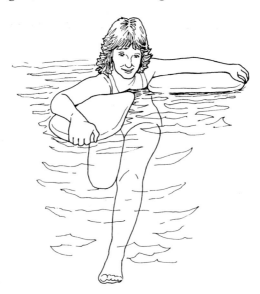

This can be slowed down to the basic movement and used to travel across the pool, or in a circle. Postnatally, this can also be developed further to include twisting with the lower body, keeping the upper torso straight. Jumps can also be incorporated postnatally. The depth of water is important for these exercises (see section on 'Teaching in small pools').

Postnatally, aerobic activities can include:

iii)   Twisting as described above, but jumping into each twist, keeping the upper torso facing forwards.

Fig. 7.4: Postnatal aerobic exercises - twists

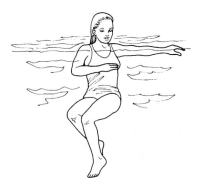

iv)   Turning. Whilst jumping, twist the upper torso around to face behind you (180°). This can lead on to jumping and turning a complete circle.

Fig. 7.5: Postnatal aerobic exercises - turning and jumping

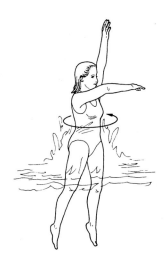

v)   Leapfrogs. Jump as if leapfrogging. This exercise can be used to travel across the pool.

vi) Star jumps. Start with legs together and jump out of the water, making a star shape with your legs and arms.

vii) Knees to chest jumps. Stretch arms above the head and jump, bringing knees to chest and arms down to knees as they come up. Reach arms up again as legs go down.

CHAPTER 8

Stretching and Cool Down

Gradually slow the speed of the aerobic section down to lead on to the stretch and cool down section.

Aims and objectives
- To stretch out the muscles and help them relax before proceeding to the cool down section.
- To return the body gradually to a calm relaxed state.
- To assist the cardiovascular system in the elimination of waste products stemming from the exercise session.
- To prepare the body for a period of relaxation.

Teaching points
Plan this section to reduce the heart rate gradually and stretch out the muscles. Work with the water, rather than against the resistance, so that the movements are smooth, slow and easy to perform.

Be aware of the women getting cold at this stage, as the body cools down quickly in water.

Examples
Stretching
A methodical pattern can be adopted working from 'top to toe' or vice versa, ensuring that all the muscles have been stretched and relaxed. The stretches should be performed slowly and sustained for 10-30 seconds, depending on the group.

The stretching exercises discussed earlier can be used or variations of them, ensuring that the head and neck, triceps and biceps, shoulders and pectorals, groin, spine, calf and hamstring, quadriceps and gluteal muscles have been stretched and relaxed.

Cool down

For the 'cool down', use any rhythmic flowing exercises, such as arm circling; arm reaching upwards and to the side; pelvic tilting and circling; pelvic floor exercises; gentle low knee lifts; partner squats; slow marching on the spot; foot circling and finally ending with a curl and stretch tall to the ceiling.

Relaxation

Using floats for support, a period of relaxation can be enjoyed by all, following an enjoyable and beneficial workout. An additional float at the ankles may help buoyancy.

Fig. 8.1: Relaxation

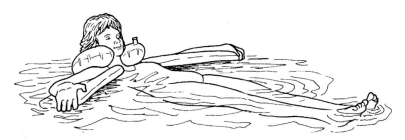

CHAPTER 9

Postnatal Notes

Classes for postnatal women have the dual advantage of the exercise session and the social support group that is frequently established and often needed at this time. The length of time following childbirth when women feel able to return to classes depends on the individual. Many things influence the decision to return, the mode of delivery, perineal trauma, vaginal loss, and the ability to be sufficiently organized to get to the pool for the session are all important factors. There are no set rules. However, perineal trauma should have healed and vaginal loss ceased before entering a pool.

The body needs time to recover after the physiological changes of pregnancy and childbirth. Ligaments are often still influenced by the hormones and remain softened for about 5-6 months. However, the immersion effect of the aquanatal sessions is quite protective to the joints, as previously discussed.

All the exercises described can be used in the postnatal session. The aerobic section can progress to a more energetic level. Abdominal exercises are especially important postnatally, as they have stretched to accommodate the growing fetus and will therefore need toning to regain their former strength. However, it is important that the rectus muscles have not separated excessively. Noble (1988) suggests that when the abdominal oblique and transverse muscles are contracted, which occurs during exercise, the separation of the straight rectus muscle increases. A distance of up to 3 cm (approximately two fingers when feeling the rectus muscle) is acceptable. Any separation greater than this increases the pressure on the linea alba and can potentially cause muscular damage. Similar care needs to be taken following a caesarean section, in view of the rectus abdominus. It is important to discuss this with the group before embarking on the abdominal exercises.

CHAPTER 10

Professional Issues

In the past, it has been asked whether midwives need to be involved with these exercise sessions. However, it is argued that midwives who have been trained to lead aquanatal exercise classes are the most appropriate and skilled professionals to take these sessions.

> A midwife is a person who ... has an important task in health counselling and education, not only for the patient, but also within the family and community. The work should involve antenatal education and preparation for parenthood.
> (A Midwife's Code of Practice, 2:1, 1991)

Aquanatal exercise classes can be seen to fulfil many of the aspects cited in this role definition of a midwife. The class is an important area in which to demonstrate healthy lifestyles and enables preparation to be made for labour. As it is an informal session, women often feel more relaxed and able to ask questions before, during, or after the session, giving them a valuable opportunity to discuss any problems that they may have.

However, the Midwife's Code of Practice also states that,

> A practising midwife must not, except in an emergency, undertake any treatment which she has not been trained to give, either before or after registration as a midwife, and which is outside her sphere of practice. (UKCC,1993).

It can be seen clearly that aquanatal sessions are well within the remit of a midwife's sphere of practice. However, it is important that adequate training has been undertaken, ensuring that the midwife is competent to plan and lead sessions (see Useful Addresses at the end of this book for details of study courses available).

Giving adequate information to the women is important. Risk-taking is a part of life and participating in exercise programmes is included in this. As suggested earlier, women can be more physically vulnerable during pregnancy, given the changes which occur within their bodies. Women should be given detailed information about this, to ensure that they make an informed choice. Those with medical or obstetric problems should be advised accordingly.

Legal aspects

There is little written about the legal aspects of midwives involved in exercise programmes. Accountability and liability appear to be the two main issues (Dimond, 1990). Gallup (1991) suggests that liability is usually based on negligence. When a midwife has failed in her duty and caused the patient harm, then she may be liable and called to account for her actions. The UKCC (1991) stipulates that a midwife's duty is to give the appropriate 'supervision, care and advice to women during pregnancy, labour and the postnatal period'. In relation to aquanatal exercises, it is important that the midwife ensures that appropriate information is given, enabling the woman to make an informed choice and the programme to be adapted to meet individual needs. Gallup (1991) suggests that failing to inform and warn clients about environmental conditions and potential dangers, may well result in liability. Ensuring both the health and safety of the woman is of paramount importance. Therefore, discussion of the safety aspects at the beginning of each class is crucial (see section on Safety aspects).

Once the appropriate information has been given, the careful planning done and sensible programmes worked out, incorporating the safety aspects mentioned, the health and safety of the women should be ensured. Sessions will then promote a healthier lifestyle and assist in a happy, healthy pregnancy. A lot of fun and enjoyment can also be shared by both the women and midwives alike, and hopefully the babies too!

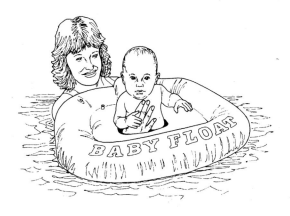

References

AMATEUR SWIMMING ASSOCIATION. (1985). *The Teaching of Swimming*. Leicester: Leicester Printers.

ARTAL, R. and ARTAL MITTLEMARK, R. (1991). 'Emotional aspects of exercise in pregnancy'. In:ARTAL MITTLEMARK, R., WISELL, R.A. and DRINKWATER, B. A. (Eds). *Exercise in Pregnancy*. Baltimore, USA:Williams and Wilkins.

ARTAL, R., MASAKI, D.I., KHODIGVIANN, N., ROMEM, Y., RUTHERFORD, S. and WISELL, R. (1989). 'Exercise prescription in pregnancy: weight bearing versus non-weight bearing'. *American Journal Of Obstetrics and Gynaecology* 161, pp.1464-69.

ARTAL MITTLEMARK, R., WISELL, R.A. and DRINKWATER, B.A. (Eds) (1991).*Exercise in Pregnancy*. Baltimore, USA:Williams and Wilkins.

BALASKAS, J. and GORDON, Y. (1990). *Water Birth*. London:Unwin Hyman.

BAUM, G. (1991). *Aquarobics*. London:Arrow Books.

BRUSER, M. (1968). 'Sporting activities during pregnancy'. *Obstetrics and Gynaecology* 32(50), pp.721-25.

COMFORT, A. (1991). *New Joy of Sex*. London:Mitchell and Beazley.

CULLUM, R. and MOWBRAY, L. (1992). *YMCA's Guide to Exercise to Music*..London:Pelham Books.

DALE, B. and ROEBER, J. (1987). *Exercise for Childbirth*. London:Century Hutchinson.

DEPARTMENT OF HEALTH (1992). *The Health of the Nation: A Strategy for health in England*. London:HMSO.

DINGWALL, R. (1993). 'Negligence litigation research and the practice of midwifery'. In: ALEXANDER, J., LEVY, V. and ROCH, S. (Eds). *Midwifery Practice: A research-based approach. Volume 4*. London:Macmillan.

DIMOND, B. (1990). *Legal Aspects of Nursing*. Hemel Hempstead:Prentice Hall/Cambridge:Cambridge University Press.

DURAK, E.P., JOVANOVIC-PETERSON, L. and PETERSON, C.M. (1990). 'Comparative evaluation of uterine response to exercise on five aerobic machines'. *American Journal of Obstetrics and Gynecology* 162(3), pp.754-56.

DRESSENDORFER, R.H. (1978). 'Physical training during pregnancy and lactation'. *Physician and Sports Medicine*, Vol. 6, pp.74-80.

EDWARDS, M.J. (1967). 'Congenital defects in guinea pigs following induced hyperthermia during gestation'. *Archives of Pathology*, Vol. 84, pp.42-44.

FLETCHER, G. (1991). *Get into Shape after Childbirth*. London:Ebury Press for the National Childbirth Trust.

GALLUP, E. (1991). 'Legal aspects of exercise prescription and pregnancy'. In: ARTAL MITTLEMARK, R., WISWELL, R.A., and DRINKWATER, B.A. (Eds). *Exercise in Pregnancy.* Baltimore, USA:Williams and Wilkins.

GILPIN, S.A., GOSLING, J.A., SMITH, A.R.B. and WARRELL, D.W. (1989). 'The pathogenesis of genitourinary prolapse and stress incontinence of urine. A histological and histochemical study'. *British Journal of Obstetrics and Gynaecology,* Vol. 96, p.15.

HARRISON, J. (1993). *Teaching Aquafit.* Sunderland:University of Sunderland.

HUCH, R. and ERKKOLA, R. (1990). 'Pregnancy and Exercise - Exercise and Pregnancy'. *British Journal of Obstetrics and Gynaecology* 61, pp. 705-9.

HUGHES, H. (1988). *The Complete Prenatal Water Workout Book.* New York, USA:Avery.

HUGHES, J.R.(1984). 'Psychological effects of habitual aerobic exercise: A critical review'. *Prev Med* Vol. 13, pp.66-78.

JOVANOVIC, L., KESSLER, A. and PETERSON, C.M. (1985). 'Human maternal and fetal response to graded exercise'. *Journal of Applied Physiology* 58, pp.1719-22.

KATZ, J. (1985). *Swimming through your Pregnancy.* Wellingborough:Thorson.

KATZ, V.L., McMURRAY, R., BERRY, M.J. and CEFALO, R.C. (1988). 'Fetal and uterine responses to immersion and exercise'. *Obstetrics and Gynaecology* 72, pp.225-30.

KATZ, V.L., McMURRAY, R. and CEFALO, R.C. (1991). 'Aquatic exercise during pregnancy'. In: ARTAL MITTLEMARK, R., WISWELL, R.A. and DRINKWATER, B.A. (Eds). *Exercise in Pregnancy.* Baltimore, USA:Williams and Wilkins.

KNUTTGEN, H.G. and EMERSON, K. (1974). 'Physiological response to pregnancy at rest and during exercise'. *Journal of Applied Physiology* Vol. 36, No. 5, pp.549-53.

KRAMER, M.S. (1992). 'Regular aerobic exercise during pregnancy'. In: ENKIN, M.W., KEIRSE, M.J.N.C., RENFREW, M.J. and NEILSON, J.P. (Eds). *Pregnancy and Childbirth Module.* Cochrane Database of Systematic Reviews: Oxford:Cochrane Updates on Disk.

KULPA, P.J., WHITE, B.M. and VISCHER, R. (1987). 'Aerobic exercise in pregnancy'. *American Journal of Obstetrics and Gynecology.,* Vol. 156, pp.1395-403.

LOTGERING, F.K., GILBERT, R.D. and LONGO, L.D.(1985). 'Maternal and fetal responses to exercise in pregnancy'. *Physiological Review* 65, pp.1-36.

LUMLEY, J. and ASTBURY, J. (1989). 'Advice for pregnancy'. In: CHALMERS, I., ENKIN, M.W. and KEIRSE, M.J.N.C. (Eds). *Effective Care In Pregnancy and Childbirth.* Oxford:Oxford University Press, pp. 237-54.

McMURRAY, R.G., KATZ, V.L., BERRY, M.J. and CEFALO, R.C. (1988). 'The effect of pregnancy on metabolic responses during rest immersion and aerobic exercise in the water'. *American Journal of Obstetrics and Gynecology* 158, pp.481-86.

McMURRAY, R.G., BERRY, M.J. and KATZ, V. (1990). 'The beta-endorphin responses of pregnant women during aerobic exercise in the water'. *Medicine and Science in Sports and Exercise* Vol. 22, No. 3, pp. 298 -303.

McMURRAY, R.G., KATZ, V.L. and MEYER-GOODWIN, W.E. (1993). 'Thermoregulation of pregnant women during aerobic exercise on land and in the water'. *American Journal of Perinatology* Vol. 10, No. 2, pp. 178-82.

MELLION, M.B. (1985). 'Exercise therapy for anxiety and depression: 1. Does the evidence justify its recommendations? 2. What are the specific considerations for clinical application?' *Postgraduate Medicine* 77(3), pp.59-98.

MILLER, P., SMITH, D.W. and SHEPHARD, T.H.E. (1978). 'Maternal hyperthermia as a possible cause of anencephally'. *Lancet* Vol. 1, pp.519-21.

MORTON, M.J., PAUL, M.S. and METCALFE, J. (1985). 'Exercise during pregnancy. Symposium on medical aspects of exercise'. *Medical Clinics of North America* 69(1), pp.97-108.

NOBLE, E. (1988). *Essential Exercise for the Childbearing Year.* Boston:Houghton Mifflin.

RAURAMO, I., ANDERSON, B. and LOATIKAIMEN, T. (1982). 'Stress hormones and placental steroids in physical exercise during pregnancy'. *British Journal of Obstetrics and Gynaecology* 89, pp.921-25.

REID CAMPION, M. (1990). *Adult Hydrotherapy: A Practical Approach.* London:Heinemann.

RUSSELL, J.B., MITCHELL, D., MUSEY, P.I. and COLLINS, D.C. (1984). 'The relationship of exercise to anovulatory cycles in female athletes: hormonal and physical characteristics'. *Obstetrics and Gynaecology* 63, pp.452-56.

RUTHERFORD, O. (1990). 'The role of exercise in prevention of osteoporosis'. *Physiotherapy,* September, Vol. 76, No. 9, pp. 522 -26.

SIBLEY, L., RUHLING, R.O., CAMERON-FOSTER, J., CHRISTENSEN, C. and BOLEN, T. (1981). 'Swimming and physical fitness during pregnancy'. *Journal of Nurse Midwifery* 26, pp.3 -12.

SONSTROEM, R.J. (1984). 'Exercise and self esteem'. *Exercise Sport Review,* Vol. 12, pp.123-55.

UNITED KINGDOM CENTRAL COUNCIL FOR NURSING, MIDWIFERY AND HEALTH VISITING (1991). *A Midwife's Code of Practice.* London:UKCC.

UNITED KINGDOM CENTRAL COUNCIL FOR NURSING, MIDWIFERY AND HEALTH VISITING (1993). *Midwives Rules.* London:UKCC.

VARRASSI, G., BUZZANO, C. and EDWARDS, T. (1989). 'Effects of physical activity on maternal plasma ß-endorphin levels and perception of labour pain'. *American Journal of Obstetrics and Gynecology* 87, pp.22-26.

WALLACE, A.M., BOYER, D.B., DAN, A. and HOLM, K. (1986). 'Aerobic exercise maternal self esteem and physical discomforts during pregnancy'. *Journal of Nurse-Midwifery* 31 (6), pp.255-61.

WALLACE, A.M. and ENGSTROM, J.L. (1987). 'The effects of aerobic exercise on the pregnant woman, fetus, and pregnancy outcome'. *Journal of Nurse-Midwifery*, Vol. 32, No. 5, pp.277-90.

WHITBY, J. (1989). *The Prenatal Exercise Book*. London:Sidgwick and Jackson.

WHITEFORD, I.H. and POLDEN, M. (1992). *Postnatal Exercises*. London:Francis Lincoln.

WILSON, N.C. and GISOLFI, C.V. (1980). 'Effects of exercising rats during pregnancy'. *Journal of Applied Physiology, Vol.* 48, pp.34-40.

WISWELL, R.A. (1991). 'Exercise physiology'. In: ARTAL MITTLEMARK, R., WISWELL, R.A. and DRINKWATER, B.A. (Eds). *Exercise in Pregnancy.* Baltimore:Williams and Wilkins.

WOLFE, L.A., HALL, P., WEBB, K.A., GOODMAN, L., MONGA, M. and McGRATH, M.J. (1989). 'Prescription of aerobic exercise during pregnancy'. *Sports Medicine* 8 (5), pp.273 - 301.

WORLD HEALTH ORGANISATION (1946). *Constitution.* Geneva:WHO.

*Biblical references taken from the Revised Standard Version of the Bible.

Further Reading

ARTAL MITTLEMARK, R., WISELL, R.A. and DRINKWATER, B.A. (Eds). (1991).*Exercise in Pregnancy.* Baltimore, USA:Williams and Wilkins.

BAUM, G. (1991). *Aquarobics.* London:Arrow Books.

HUGHES, H. (1988). *The Complete Prenatal Water Workout Book.* New York:Avery.

REED, B. and MURRAY, R. (1985). *Water Workout.* Australia:Sun Books.

Useful Addresses

Equipment

Swim Shop, 52/58 Albert Road, Luton, Beds, LU1 3PR. Tel: 0582 416545. (Other mail order companies advertised in any swimming journal.)

Video and books

ASA Swimming Enterprises, Harold Ferhouse, Derby Square, Loughborough, Leics, LE11 0AL.

Floats used for relaxation

Catalogue no. L8292-5, Nottingham Rehab Ltd., Ludlow Hill Road, West Bridgford, Notts, NG2 6HD. Tel: 0602 452345.

Courses

NCT (ask for events list), Alexandria House, Oldham Terrace, Acton, London W3 6NH. Tel: 081 992 8637.

Aquarobics, 143 White Hart Lane, Barnes, London SW13 0JP. Tel: 081 878 9868.

Other courses are advertised in the midwifery journals.

Index

R

rectus muscle 41, 53
relaxation
  8, 15, 17, 21, 22, 51, 52
resistance
  7, 9, 15, 18, 19, 20, 37, 39, 51
rotation of spine 26, 40

S

safety aspects 16, 55
shoulders 25, 51
size of class 18
small pools 18-19
spine 25, 51
staffing levels 18
stamina 5, 8, 9, 21, 37, 38, 46
static stretches 21, 30-36
stretch reflex 30
stretching exercises 24, 51
structure. *See* classes: structure
supervisor of midwives 10

T

teaching in small pools 18-19
teaching points. *See* classes:
  teaching points
temperature
 body 5, 9, 17, 21, 24
 optimum 13
 water 13, 18
thighs 44
triceps 37, 38, 39, 51
twists 41, 42, 49

U

UKCC documents 54, 55
upper spine 25

V

valsalva effect 22
voice projection 19

W

waist exercises 28
warm-up 21, 24-29
water resistance. *See* resistance
wrists 28